Beginner's Nutrition Guide

TO ENHANCE SPORT PERFORMANCE, HEALTHY LIFESTYLE, AND WEIGHT LOSS

By: Von Bailey

Table of Contents

Nutrition at A Glance

What is Nutrition?

Nutrition can be defined as the process of giving the body food that is required for proper health and growth. Nutrition is nourishment for the body in the form of food. From a scientific aspect, nutrition is the science that refers to nutrients and nutrition within the human body.

Why is Nutrition Important?

Nutrition is essential for many different reasons. The primary reason nutrition is important is because it is required for a balanced diet. A balanced diet is needed for overall health and wellbeing. Without nutrition, the human body cannot function properly. A wide range of foods are necessary to give the human body proper nutrition.

Components of Nutrition

There are six components of nutrition that include, protein, carbohydrates, fats, vitamins, minerals and water. Here are reasons these components are essential.

1. **Protein**- Protein is found in every fiber of the human body, such as hair and nails. Protein helps the body heal by building and repairing tissue. This component of nutrition is required for the creation of essential body chemicals, including hormones and enzymes. Without protein, skin, bones, muscles and blood would encounter many issues.
2. **Carbohydrates**- Carbohydrates are required to create energy in the human body. Carbohydrates are found in many vegetable, dairy, bread, fruit and pasta products. Carbohydrates aid with the creation of glucose. Glucose is required for the creation of energy.
3. **Fats**- A lot of people are under the impression that fats are bad. All fats do not have a negative impact on the human body. In fact, fat is responsible for Omega 3. Omega 3 is an essential fat because it cannot be created by the human body like other components of nutrition. Fats are needed to help the body absorb A, D, and E vitamins.
4. **Vitamins**- Vitamins and minerals work together to perform many beneficial functions for the body. Vitamins help the body heal its wounds and boost the immune system. Vitamins assist the body with energy creation and repairing cellular damage.
5. **Minerals**- Minerals are essential for nutrition and proper bodily functions. Minerals are important for the skin, hair, muscles, nerve function and forming strong bones. Minerals help with metabolic functions that help convert energy into food.
6. **Water**- Water is the universal solvent for the entire human body and one of the most important substances in the world. Water helps everything from plants, animals and everything else that exist in the world survive and thrive. Water hydrates the human body and acts as a lubricant during the digestion process. The human body can survive without food longer than it can without water.

Whether you are an athlete, teenager or a person who is considered overweight and wants to lead a healthier lifestyle, nutrition is the key to success. Great nutrition helps athletes perform better, helps teenagers with healthy growth and posture and helps people who are overweight eat healthier and reach a healthy weight.

Nutrition for Athletes

Athletes require nutrition to keep their bodies functioning properly. Athletes demand a lot from their body and require more calories than a person who is not as active as an athlete. Here are a few things athletes require for nutrition.

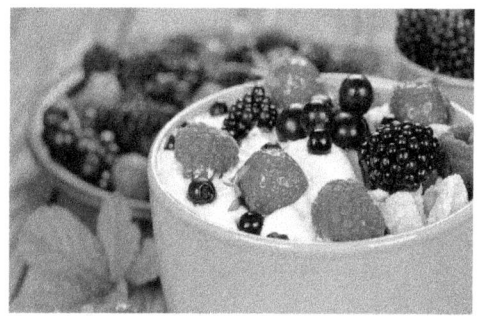

Energy

Energy- Energy for an athlete is requires a constant supply of carbohydrates. Other sources of energy include fat, protein, carbohydrates, minerals and vitamins. There are many different components of energy which includes basic metabolic needs, growth, temperature regulation and physical activity. These instances are the essentials of energy. An athlete's body demands the essentials of energy on a daily basis, so their diet must reflect their requirements to meet the needs of the essential functions.

Energy Balance is a term used to describe the met requirements of an athlete's daily intake. The daily intake is food energy that derives from protein, carbohydrates, alcohol and fat. When the daily intake is equal to the daily intake of the energy expenditure, it is referred to as energy balance. The equation for energy balance is:

- Energy Balance= energy intake-energy expenditure

Another aspect of energy is energy availability. Energy availability is the amount of remaining energy that can contribute to the human body's physiological requirements.

Eating Frequency

Athletes must maintain an eating frequency so their nutritional demands are met. Here are the steps that are required for a balanced meal, diet routine for an athlete to perform better.

1. **Start in the Right Direction**
   Breakfast will always be the most essential meal of the day. An athlete's breakfast should consist of fruit, yogurt and other foods that are nutrient-rich.

2. **Devise a Plan**
   Training is an important part of an athlete's life, but eating is more important. When you plan ahead, make sure you have enough performance foods for a reliable, balanced source of energy. Performance food should be consumed every two to three hours. These foods can be eaten between meals and while you are training.

3. **Make Necessary Changes**

When you make the necessary changes, it may be difficult at first to stick to a routine and get your body used to the changes you have made. The good news is it gets better. As time passes, your body will adjust to the changes you have made.

4. **Keep Energy During Training**

Training takes a toll on your body and your body requires an ample amount of energy and nutrition. Proper nutrition and a reliable energy source are required for a successful training session. Training sessions can be long or short. Sessions that last longer than 60 minutes take a terrible toll on your body and consumes a lot of energy. When training sessions are one hour or more, you will need to consume a snack that is rich in carbohydrates. If you prefer a beverage over a snack, choose a beverage that is high in carbohydrates. Sports drinks are the perfect beverage to consume during training because it replenishes things that are lost during training, including electrolytes and fluid. Foods that are great for training include sports bars, bread with jelly, bananas, granola and dried fruit. Although drinking water seems like a good idea, when you are consuming carbohydrates, water should be avoided because it can cause problems with your stomach.

5. **Refueling Your Body**

Your body runs out of energy like a steam engine runs out of coal or a battery dies in a remote. As an athlete, it is important to replace the energy you use. Here are a few things you can do to replenish your energy. You should plan to have one meal within one hour of your training. This meal should include foods that are high in protein and full of carbohydrates. You need an adequate amount of water or other beverage that satisfies your thirst and replenishes electrolytes and other things your body loses during training. Your body may require a recovery snack. This snack needs to be consumed within half an hour of training. A recovery snack is critical when you have more than one training session scheduled. Recovery nutrition is a part of refueling your body. Recovery nutrition foods and beverages include low-fat chocolate milk, fruit smoothies, trail mix, yogurt parfaits and cereal and milk.

Nutrition Meal Plans for Athletes

Every athlete wants to perform at their best. In order for the best performance, athletes need to have a healthy diet. Athletes need to have a healthy diet. Athletes require a well-balanced diet that includes healthy fats, protein, carbohydrates and vitamins. Although athletes must consume more food than people who are not athletes, their food choices must be healthy and wholesome. Athletes must consume between 2,000 to 5,000 calories on a daily basis.

Breakfast

Breakfast for an athlete needs to consist of an abundance of protein and carbohydrates. Your body needs fuel to revamp itself from the previous night's sleep. Great foods to consume for breakfast include turkey bacon, skim milk, fruit, soy products, eggs and whole grain cereals. Eating a wholesome breakfast will give you a boost of energy and an abundance of fuel for the day.

Lunch

Low-calorie meals are best for lunch for athletes. Low-calorie meals consist of a lot of fruits and vegetables. Light pasta dishes are great for lunch.

Dinner

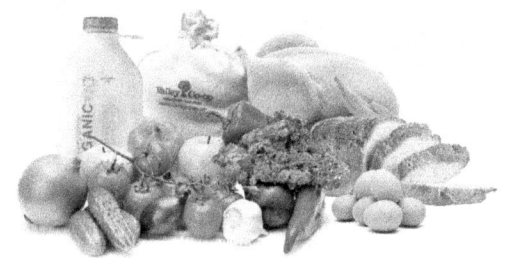

Dinner is the final meal of the day. You don't need to overdo it by piling various foods on your plate. Dinner should consist of a meal that is full of healthy, fatty foods, carbohydrates, vitamins, fiber and protein. This is an example of a well-balanced dinner. Different foods you could consume include whole-wheat bread chicken breasts, green beans and whole-wheat rice. As for dessert, fresh fruit is an excellent option.

Recipes for Breakfast, Lunch and Diner

Breakfast

Avocado Toast with Egg

Avocado toast with egg is a simple, yet nutritious breakfast meal.

Ingredients

- *1 ready (ripe) avocado*
- *1 teaspoon fresh lemon juice*
- *Sprinkle of sea salt*
- *Dash of fresh ground pepper*
- *2 whole large eggs cooked sunny side up*
- *2 pieces of toast (use multi-grain bread)*

- ○ *Optional Ingredients*
- *Black beans*
- *Sliced tomatoes*
- *Fresh shredded cheddar cheese*

Instructions

1. *Toast both slices of multi-grain bread to your liking.*
2. *Lengthwise, cut the avocado in half. To perfectly separate the avocadoes, twist them, then proceed with removing the pit.*
3. *Throw the avocado pit away and scoop out the inside of the avocado with a spoon.*
4. *Place the scooped insides of the avocado in a small to medium-sized bowl. Mash the insides of the avocado together using a fork. Once the insides are mushy, add the lemon juice and stir until they are thoroughly mixed together.*
5. *Cook your eggs fluffy and sunny side up.*
6. *Gently spread the avocado and lemon juice mixture on your toast evenly or to your liking on both pieces of toast.*
7. *Place one egg on each piece of toast. Sprinkle and dash ground pepper and sea salt, tomatoes, cheese and any other toppings you desire on the egg and toast.*
8. *Put both pieces of toast together to make a sandwich or consume them individually. Enjoy with juice or water.*

Peanut Butter Banana Smoothie

A peanut butter banana smoothie is the perfect way to begin your day. It is full of protein and other essentials you need for a boost of energy that will help get you through the day. This smoothie can be a great breakfast meal or healthy snack for in between meals.

Ingredients

- 2 tablespoons creamy peanut butter
- 1 cup pure almond milk
- 5-6 whole ice cubes

Instructions

1. *Place the peanut butter, almond milk and ice cubes in a blender.*

2. *Blend the mixture on high until it is smooth or to your liking and enjoy.*

Lunch

Kale and Apple Salad

This salad takes your taste buds on a journey it will never forget while providing the proper nutrients and vitamins for powerful, long-lasting energy. Kale is rich in antioxidants and combines the taste of many different flavors from dates, cheese, apples and almonds. This salad is a light meal that will satisfy your hunger.

Ingredients

- *3 tablespoons of pure fresh lemon juice*
- *2 tablespoons of pure extra-virgin olive oil*
- *Fresh kosher salt*
- *1 bunch fresh kale (remove ribs-slice leaves thin)*
- *¼ cup fresh dates*
- *1 whole honey crisp apple*
- *¼ cup toasted, slivered almonds*
- *1 ounce finely grated pecorino*
- *Fresh ground black pepper*

Instructions

1. *In a large mixing bowl, using a whisk, mix ¼ teaspoons of kosher salt, lemon juice and olive oil together until thoroughly mixed.*
2. *Add kale and stir around in mixture until the kale is coated. Let kale marinate for 10 minutes.*
3. *Slice dates into thin slivers*
4. *Cut apple into long, thin slices (apples should look like match sticks)*
5. *Place sliced dates and cut apples into a medium-sized bowl with almonds and cheese. Season blend with a sprinkle of kosher salt and fresh ground pepper. Mix thoroughly. Grab a fork and enjoy.*

Vegetable Pocket Stacks

A pita pocket stack is more nutritious than a hot pocket for an athlete any day. This wholesome meal is a great alternative to old cuts and packs a lot of vitamins and nutrition.

Ingredients

- *(1) 15-ounce can of white beans or chickpeas (drained)*
- *1 ½ tablespoons of water*
- *¼ cup fresh grated pecorino cheese or fresh Romano cheese*
- *2 tablespoons of fresh lemon juice*
- *1 teaspoon kosher salt*
- *Sprinkle of red pepper flakes*
- *¼ cup extra-virgin olive oil*
- *Fresh ground black pepper*
- *Pitted and sliced ½ ripe avocado*
- *1 sliced fresh small cucumber (bell pepper can be used as an alternative-seeds removed and sliced)*
- *10-12 lightly toasted mini pita breads*

Instructions

1. Gently mix lemon juice, red pepper flakes, water, chickpeas and cheese in a food processor. A blender can be used, but only on its lowest setting. The mixture needs to be completely smooth. Blend more if lumps are present.
2. Pour olive oil in blender or food processor while mixing it on low power. When complete, the mixture should appear smooth and have a Velvet texture. Use pepper to season to your liking.
3. Scoop a few tablespoons of bean spread onto the toasted pitas. If there is bean spread left over, store it in an air-tight container to use later.
4. On top of the bean spread, place cucumber slices and avocados. Other vegetables of your choice can be added. Season the vegetables to your liking and enjoy your meal!

Dinner

Oven-Baked Salmon

Oven-baked salmon is the perfect nutritious meal for a busy week or weekend. You don't have to go above and beyond to get proper nutrition.

Ingredients

- 12-ounce salmon fillet (cut into 4 pieces)
- Salt (course-grain)
- Fresh ground black pepper
- Toasted almond parsley salsa (for serving purposes)
- Baked squash (optional)
- Toasted parsley almond salad

Toasted Parsley Almond Salad

- 1 fresh shallot
- 1 tablespoon of red wine vinegar
- Salt (course-grain)
- 2 tablespoons of rinsed capers
- 1 cup flat-leaf parsley (fresh)
- ½ cup toasted almonds
- Extra-virgin olive oil

Instructions

1. Preheat oven to 450 degrees Fahrenheit
2. Season salmon with a dash of salt and pepper
3. Place salmon skin side down, on a non-stick pan or foil so salmon will not stick and tear apart
4. Thoroughly cook salmon (approx. 13-15 minutes)
5. Salmon can be served with toasted almond parsley salad if desired

Toasted Almond Parsley Salad

1. Mince shallot and place in small bowl
2. Mix vinegar and a dash of salt to the shallots and let marinate for 25-30 minutes
3. Roughly chop parsley, almonds and capers before adding to the shallot mixture. Add olive oil to taste

Zesty Shrimp Scampi

Shrimp scampi, as many people know it, is full of buttery goodness, but zesty shrimp scampi is a lighter meal option that bursts with flavor.

Ingredients

- *6 ounces spaghetti (multi-grain)*
- *¼ cup crushed fresh multi-grain croutons*
- *¼ cup chopped fresh leaf parsley (flat leaf)*
- *1 ½ tablespoons of fresh grated lemon zest*
- *1 tablespoon virgin olive oil*
- *1 thinly sliced fresh shallot*
- *1 minced garlic clove*
- *¼ teaspoon crushed red pepper*
- *16 fresh large shrimp or 21-25 small shrimp (both shelled and deveined)*
- *¼ teaspoon salt*
- *¼ cup low-sodium chicken broth*
- *¼ cup white wine (dry)*
- *1 tablespoon fresh lemon juice*
- *1 tablespoon black, pitted, chopped olives (black)*

Instructions

1. Place half-full pot of water on the stove over medium heat. Bring to a boil and add pasta. Allow pasta to cook for 7-10 minutes. When the pasta is done, drain and set to the side.
2. In a small bowl, combine, then mix, ½ tablespoon of parsley, croutons and 1 tablespoon of zest. Once mixed, set aside.
3. Using a large non-stick skillet, pour a generous amount of oil in the pan. Turn stove on medium and allow oil to heat.
4. When oil is warm, add garlic, red pepper and shallot. Stir mixture every 10-15 seconds until shallots are soft. This should take about 1 minute.
5. Once the shallots are soft, add shrimp and salt. Cook over medium-high heat. While cooking, turn the shrimp every 15-20 seconds until they are opaque.
6. Mix in olives, broth, lemon juice and wine. Bring the contents in the skillet to a boil, let mixture cook for 1 minute, then decrease heat to medium.
7. Mix in spaghetti parsley and zest. Mix ingredients thoroughly to give food coating. Remove from heat and place skillet contents in a large bowl. Sprinkle with croutons and enjoy!

15 Foods Athletes Should Eat for Nutrition

There are a few foods all athletes should eat in the days before an occasion to guarantee top performance. Here are 15 Foods Athletes Should Eat for Nutrition

1. **Entire grains**-entire grain sustenance, for example, oat, bagels, pasta, and bread give good, long-enduring vitality to the entire body. As the most critical nutrition type, athletes should eat many entire grain sugars before an event.

2. **Nutty spread**-nutty spread is a decent wellspring of protein and fundamental fats, and it is anything but difficult to convey and eat on the go. Other protein sources will function too, for example, incline meat or dairy; the vital thing is to get satisfactory protein before and after a workout. Protein helps the body in keeping up oxygen consuming digestion system rather than anaerobic digestion system, which keeps the body from taking protein from incline tissue. Sufficient protein speeds recuperation and aides in genuine performance circumstances.

3. **New products of the soil**-is a great approach to get vitamins and minerals that offer the body some assistance with functioning as would be expected. They are generally without fat and contain loads of vitality for the body to use amid activity. A few natural products, for example, bananas, contain potassium, a mineral that directs water levels in the body and balances out muscle compression. Low potassium levels can prompt muscle issues and weariness, so eating potassium-rich foods is a smart thought.

4. **Calcium-Rich Foods**-foods, for example, cheddar, yogurt, and milk contain essential calcium, which creates solid bones and shields athletes from damage.

5. **Fiber-Rich Foods**-Fiber is the nutritional part that keeps athletes full and controls the digestive tract. Many of the foods as of now specified incorporate fiber, however it is critical for mentors to know which foods offer athletes some assistance with regulating fiber levels.

6.**Non-wheat pasta** - Wheat is by and large bravo. It gives fiber and moderate smoldering complex sugars. In any case, many wheat items have gluten, a protein that can bring about genuine digestive wellbeing issues.

7.**Milk** - It has casein protein, which is a slower processing protein. This implies you will have a steadier stream of vitality contrasted with when drinking things stacked with basic sugars, for example, organic product juices, which have a sensational drop in vitality after a starting spike.

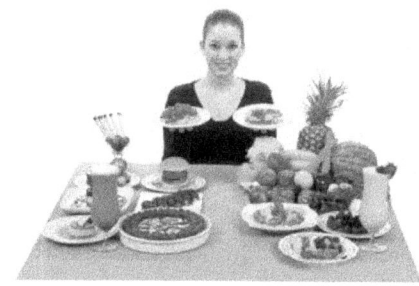

8.**Apples** - The skins in apples contain a substance called quercetin, a characteristic vitality promoter.

9.**Coffee** - There are various studies demonstrating that devouring moderate measures of juiced drinks undoubtedly increment athletic performance.

10.**Kale**-Have a go at swapping out your spinach for kale. Kale is more supplement thick than spinach, offering more calcium, vitamin A, vitamin C, and more cancer prevention agents.

11. **Sweet Potatoes and Yams**-Sweet potatoes are the ideal recuperation nourishment.

12. **Coconut**-Coconut contains medium-chain triglycerides. MCTs are all the more quickly consumed by the body and can be blazed as fuel snappier than different forms of fat, making them a feasible wellspring of vitality amid activity.

13. **Eggs**-Athletes love grain, yet changing to eggs for breakfast can have some key advantages, including giving more protein and fat than a dish of oat and keeping you full more.

14. **Sardines**-Yes, I said sardines! These little folks are a nutrition power-house! They offer a huge amount of Omega 3 fats while being sheltered from mercury due to their little size.

15 **Meat**-Do you eat enough protein? Continuance athletes need somewhere around 1.2 and 2.0 grams of protein for each pound of body weight each day.

Nutrition for Teens

Many people want to know about nutrition for teens. It is a little different from the nutrition that is required for an athlete or an adult. Teens require a wider variety of food than adults because of how active they are. When you are active, you require more food to help replace energy you lose.

THE NUTRITIONAL NEEDS OF A TEENAGER

As teens grow, they will experience appetite surges. The appetite surge generally occurs by age 10 for girls and age 12 for boys. Most of the time, this is the appetite surge right before the growth spurt of puberty occurs. For a teenager, calories are used to express the amount of energy that is delivered by food. Adolescence is the time when the most food is required. An adolescent boy requires 2,800 calories per day. An adolescent girl requires 2,200 calories per day.

Nutrients and Nutrition

When it comes to having energy, a teenager's body requires healthy fats, protein and carbohydrates. Each gram of carbohydrate or protein supplies the body with as many as 4 calories Healthy fats contribute as many as 9 calories for every gram consumed.

Protein

Protein is important, but it is not as essential as other nutrients because teenagers receive two times the amount of protein they require.

Great sources of protein for a teenager include:

- Beef
- Turkey
- Cheese
- Chicken
- Eggs
- Pork
- Fish

Carbohydrates

Carbohydrates for a teenager can be complex to understand. Carbohydrates are commonly found in sugars and starches. Glucose is the teenager's body's main fuel source and it derives from carbohydrates. Although all carbohydrates are not equal, teens should consume as many foods that contain complex carbohydrates as possible. Teenagers do not need to stay away from simple carbohydrates, but they should consume them in moderation. Simple carbohydrates provide a teenager's body with bursts of energy, but unlike complex-carbohydrates, the energy is not sustained.

Dietary Fats

Fats should account for no more than 30 percent of a teenager's diet. Fat within the diet is important because it helps the body in many different ways, including absorbing fat-soluble vitamins (A, E, D, and K), and supplying the body with energy. Teenagers who partake in a diet that is heavy in fats will gain a substantial amount of weight whether the teen is active or not. Why? All fatty foods contain cholesterol. This wax-like substance can clog arteries and cause other serious health problems.

Dietary fats are divided into three proportions, which include saturated, polyunsaturated and monounsaturated fats.

Saturated Fats: These fats can be found in many different foods, including palm oil, butter, cheese, pork, egg yolks, lamb, cream and coconut oil.

Polyunsaturated Fats: These fats are found in many different types of oil, including sesame see, corn, safflower, soybean, cottonseed and sunflower oil.

Monounsaturated Fats: This type of fat is the healthiest out of the three types of fats. Monounsaturated fats can be found in canola oil, olives, olive oil, peanut butter, walnuts, walnut oil, peanuts, peanut oil and cashews.

Vitamins and Minerals

A diet that is well-rounded and balanced requires vitamins and minerals. A balanced diet must include all of the essential vitamins and mineral. Teenagers should focus their attention on their daily requirements of Vitamin D, calcium, zinc and iron because these are the vitamins and minerals they often do not meet the requirements for.

In the fast food age, almost everyone's diet is lacking somewhere and teenagers are probably the worst. In the fast food age, junk is more abundant, easier and even cheaper than the foods that they need to better maintain their health.

A lack of nutrients can lead to serious complications even for teens and prolonged deficiencies can affect them later in life. From causing anemia and lowered immune system function right now, to affecting their bones, hearts and minds the eating habits of teens are tearing them down overall.

1. **Nuts-** Salty, crunchy, good for you! Nuts are an effective nutrient dense snack that can be used to replace some go to junk for teens and adults alike.

2. **Avocados-** Diet fads sweep through high school and anyone who remembers going knows the low-fat is on the list. Those who aren't worried about dieting though are eating a diet high in saturated fats. Avocados however offer unsaturated fats (the good kind) and Vitamin E.

3. **Dark lettuces-** Spinach, kale, and even romaine are all a step up from the iceberg stand by. Antioxidants and iron found in these varieties boost energy levels and strengthen immune systems.

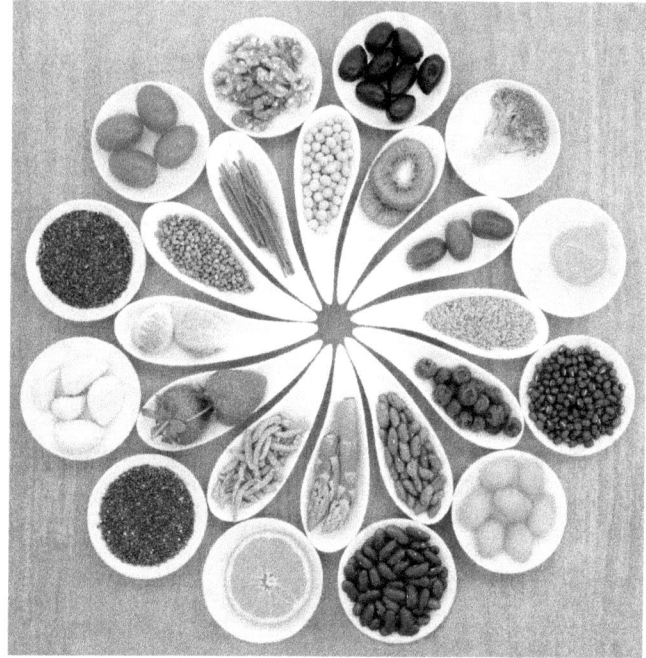

4. **Red meat-** Iron deficiencies in teenage girls runs rampant! Replacing the iron they lose every month is crucial to proper development and health.

5. **Cheese-** Calcium builds bones and theirs are still developing

6. **Yogurt-** Calcium helps protect their bones while live and active probiotics found in most yogurt keeps their digestive

system running smooth.

7. **Oily fish-** Omega 3's and healthy fats found in oily fish like salmon and mackerel help build a still developing brain and aid in the absorption of vital vitamins and nutrients.

8. **Fruits-** There is a range of vitamins and minerals missing from the modern Western diet, fruit whether, fresh or dried can help make up the gap between what teens do eat and what they need.

9. **Berries-** On the list of super foods that boost overall health. From Alzheimer's to heart disease and everything in between, berries are simple portable food that fights it off.

10. **Broccoli-** Cliché as it sounds, teens need to eat their broccoli. Broccoli is dense in protein, helps lower cholesterol and fight inflammation.

11. **Tomatoes-** One of the best place to find lycopene which can help fights off cancer.

12. **Whole Grain Breads-** Replacing refined grains with whole grains leads to better blood sugar levels and better moods. Decreasing risk of future complications including diabetes.

13. **Smoothies-** Pack in a real breakfast! Ditch the Pop-tarts and pile in fruits, vegetables and low-fat milk into a blender to get a teen's day started on the right foot.

14. **Water-** Proper hydration is key to everything from appetite regulation to brain function. 8 glasses a day is recommended.

15. **Chocolate-** Not the cheap sugary fake stuff, but a little dark, rich chocolate can provide a teen with enough zinc to stay healthy and strong.

The sooner a teen can get their diet on the right track the more likely their eating habits will stick and translate into a healthy lifestyle that follows them through life. Nutrition is connected to health, performance and success!

Nutritional Requirement for Teenagers

Food is the main source of nutrition for teenagers. It acts as a fuel for the growing as well as developing children. From this phase a child gradually develops lifetime food habits. Every parents more or less can offer healthy diets to their children during their teenage years. During teenage days, a complete physical changes occurs during the time of puberty. At this stage a greater amount of nutrition is required for the teenagers in comparison with adults or young who have completed their growing phase.

Main nutrients for the teenagers include:

Calcium: Calcium is obtained mainly in the dairy foods. Good amount of dairy foods can be given during adolescence which results in developing strong bone density.

Iron: For developing blood volume and muscle mass, iron rich foods are required for the teenagers. Additional iron is also required for girls because of their periods. Among all foods, red meat is one of the main source of iron which can be taken in their daily nutrition. Green leafy vegetables, beans, lentils, grains and cereals also contains high percentage of iron.

Vitamins and Minerals: For proper growth and development a child needs a good amount of essential vitamins and minerals. It generally includes Vitamins A, B, C, D, E and minerals such as zinc, iodine, calcium and iron. Foods which contains vitamins and minerals are:

- Vegetables
- Bread
- Pasta
- Rice
- Corn
- Milk
- Cheese
- Curd
- Yogurt
- Egg
- Chicken
- Meat
- Legumes (High in protein)

Different ways of nutrition for teenagers are given below (Breakfast to Dinner):

Breakfast: milk, eggs, carrots, fruits (rich in Vitamin A) - Helps in developing immunity, good eyesight, skin and cheese, breads, yeast extracts (rich in Vitamin B1) - Helps in the gradual breakdown of fats, proteins and carbohydrates.

Lunch: rice, cereals, meat, fish, eggs, chicken, legumes, vegetables, curd. Carbohydrate intake is a necessity for all teenagers for muscle development. Vitamin C fruits can also be taken, such as citrus, kiwi which results in developing strong teeth and gums. Leafy green vegetables, liver and some wholegrain cereals contain folic acid which are beneficial for protein absorption resulting in the formation of new blood cells and DNA.

Dinner: rice, wholegrain cereals, milk, fish, meat, eggs, chicken can be consumed. Breads can be

consumed instead of rice.
Different ways to promote healthy teenage eating habits:

1. Instead of focusing on specific foods, the focus of overall diet is required.

2. Homemade foods are far healthier and hygienic. Restaurant and fast food / processed foods contains unhealthy fat, sugar and salt which is not beneficial for health.

3. A variety of healthy snacks are better than empty calorie snack.

One of the best things to remember about maintaining a healthy diet is to eat a large array of foods. There is no one food in the world that exists that is able to supply all of the necessary nutrition that adults require. The famous food pyramids are most certainly a recommended reference in order to follow a scientifically proven mode of consuming the needed nutrients. The tip of the pyramid are the foods that are discretionary and left to the individual person to choose what to eat, while the base is what is highlighted as the most important. It is imperative for the readers to recall that a balanced diet is paramount, and that too much of anything will result in a negative outcome – regardless if it's considered healthy.

The energy needed to keep functioning throughout the day unsurprisingly comes from the nutrition that adults gather from eating plentiful and well spread out meals. Most of the energy comes from carbohydrates that we eat, which is found in both starch and sugars. If necessary, our energy also comes from stored fats in our bodies. However, containing the energy within our body without burning any calories will result in the carbohydrates being stored in the previously mentioned fats in our bodies – resulting in weight gain.

This leads us to the conclusion that exercise is an important part of the routine to keep us in 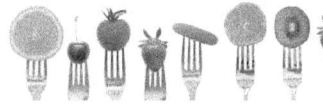 shape. There are plenty of ways that people choose to exercise: for example, playing sports such as football, soccer, volleyball, figure skating, hockey, and gymnastics among countless others. Running or taking a walk around the neighborhood is perfectly sufficient as well – just as long as you're getting a minimum of thirty minutes of physical activity per day. If you dislike the outdoors and prefer to stay healthy on your own, there is always the use of technology. Games on platforms such as Wii Fit on the Wii or the Just Dance is a wonderful way to burn some calories without having to leave the comfort of your own home if that just isn't for you.

Another added bonus to eating three healthy meals a day, drinking plenty of fluids, and physical activities will lead to a regulated sleep schedule. After going throughout your work day and exercising, general tiredness and exhaustion will settle in during the evening. This is the time to relax in your favorite reclining chair and unwind. As you are tired, you're more likely to fall asleep and wake up around the same time – leaving you ready to face the new day's challenges with a well-rested and positive attitude.

Great Food Sources for Nutrition for Adults

Nutrition for adults is not to be taken lightly. After discussing all of the ways that will contribute to keeping a healthy mind and body, it's time to examine the types of nutrients and foods that will be the best for us.

Human beings are comprised of 70% water, just as the Earth is covered mostly in bodies of water. This means that drinking fluids – especially plain water itself – are absolutely necessary for staying healthy. Three glasses of water are the suggested intake each day. Dehydration can easily lead to multiple physical pains such as headaches, stomachaches, diarrhea, and more.

Protein is a critical nutrient for the regulation of the human being's body. It helps in regulating skin, hair, nails, and the lean mass of the body. It's recommended that adults on average require 46 to 56 grams of protein daily; however, if you are particularly active and a frequent exerciser, then some more might be a benefit in the long run for you. Foods that contain this nutrient include poultry, fish, eggs, dairy food, soy foods, and nuts. Some examples of individual foods that are recommended include 2% milk, Greek yogurt, cottage cheese, steak, chicken, and turkey. Zinc can also be found in these foods, especially in seafood.

Dairy products and vegetables that are known to be green and leafy will help provide your daily amount of calcium. Your calcium intake is extremely important, as it is what creates and helps to maintain our bodies. Our bones and teeth in particular are comprised of calcium. The suggested amount of intake for calcium is approximately 1,000 to 1,200 milligrams per each day. Food that have calcium include dairy products, vegetables, and cereals. A few examples of specific foods include, milk, spinach, broccoli, cheese, yogurt, brand-name cereals, and orange juice. Iron can also be found in a majority of these foods.

As mentioned before, carbohydrates are the source of our energy to complete activities on a daily basis. Although they're found in sugars, carbohydrates are also present in a variety of starches such as bread and rice. Fruits are also good if one is searching for a healthier snack. It is recommended that people consume their carbs from starches like grains, instead of sugars which should be reserved for the infrequent treat.

Nutrients for adults are absolutely necessary; not only for maintaining a healthy body, but also a healthy mind. Many people's mental health are affected by the state of their body and if they're not eating well. If you are being burdened by stress or anxiety, perhaps eating a balanced meal with assist you in feeling better. Exercise requires energy to complete, and physical activity as well has been proven to help calm people in times of distress. In addition to maintaining a healthy body for ourselves, we are acting as role models for our children and the younger generations. Even though vegetables may not taste the best, they're still vital to our well-being – and that is a lesson from childhood that will stick with us for the rest of our lives.

The natural aging process is something no one can avoid.

Some of us resort to drastic measures like surgery, but if you're more pragmatic in your approach, you know and understand an active lifestyle with a solid dieting plan can make all the difference.

A wide spectrum of change occurs in the human body as we age if we don't take care of ourselves.

Our skin produces less natural skin oil which can result in dry, itchy, damaged skin. As a result, wrinkles, age spots, skin tags become more prominent. Our bones typically lose density and strength, shrink in size, which makes them more prone to fractures. Our muscle mass generally shrinks and we become weaker, and a host of other things.

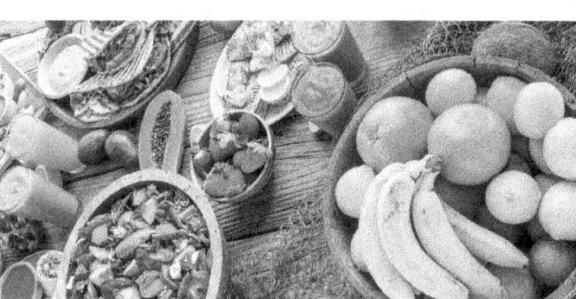

This is natural, but we can soften the blow with a strong diet.

1.Oats

A steaming hot bowl of oatmeal is perhaps one of the healthiest ways to start your day. Oats are packed with fiber and just one cup packs 10grams of protein. Oats are also rich in calcium and potassium, which are known to reduce blood pressure.

2.Apples

On top of being one of the most recognizable brand labels ever, apples are incredibly rich in antioxidants, flavonoids, and dietary fiber. The antioxidants in apples may help reduce developing cancer, hyper tension, heart disease, and diabetes.

3.Quinoa

Quinoa is a little known secret amongst health enthusiasts and professionals. Known as one of the most protein rich foods we consume, Quinoa is packed with iron, lysine, and magnesium. If you aren't a meat eater, this food should serve as an excellent substitute.

4.Nuts

All nuts have varying nutritional credentials and will offer various health benefits. Almonds for example, are rich in calcium and are ideal for those of us who can't consume dairy products. Brazil nuts assist with low thyroid function, and cashews contribute a good level of protein and are a useful source of minerals like iron and zinc.

5.Kale

One cup of kale is only 33 calories, but you get so much! Three grams of protein, 2.5 grams of fiber, vitamins A, C, and K, Folate, a B vitamin that's key for brain development, and alpha-linolenic acid, and omega 3 fatty acid. If you search up a list of "Super Foods," kale is usually near the top

6.Potatoes

Can you believe that potatoes were thought to be poisonous at one point in history? Thankfully that is no longer the case so we can enjoy one of the most popular foods around. Potatoes are action packed with health benefits: calcium, magnesium, zing and potassium for bone health and blood health. Fiber, vitamin C, and vitamin B-6 for heart health. We could go on and on. It is said that you can live up to 30 years on nothing but potatoes.

7.Berries

Strawberries, blueberries, and blackberries are powerful superfoods. The list of nutrients packed in them are so vast that we could write an entire post on berries alone. The anti-oxidants and phytochemicals may help prevent (and in some cases reverse) the effects of aging, cardiovascular disease, arthritis, diabetes, high blood pressure and certain types of cancer.

8.Cinnamon

Cinnamon is one of the most delicious, healthiest spices in existence and is high in substance with powerful medicinal properties. It can lower blood sugar levels, cut the risk of heart disease, and can improve sensitivity to the hormone insulin, which helps regulate metabolism and energy use.

9.Yogurt

Yogurt, simultaneously overrated and underrated, has a host of health benefits that will not only improve your bodily function, but your actual appearance. Eat 18 ounces a day and you can drop a jean size. Most brands of yoga contain good-for-you bacteria that strengthens your immune system.

10.Fish

Fish is a classic staple of a healthy diet. A high-protein, low-fat food that provides a diverse range of health benefits, there are entire cultures on the planet that survive on fish and just fish alone. Fish are high in omega-3 fatty acids which improve your circulation and heart health.

11.Broccoli

Nothing strikes fear in the hearts of children more at the dinner table then a stalk of broccoli. Luckily, most of us grew out of that phase and can appreciate all the things broccoli does for our digestive, immune, and cardiovascular systems. This vegetable is a powerhouse of nutrients and even has cancer preventing properties.

12. Dark Chocolate

Dark chocolate is loaded with nutrients that can positively affect your health. Made from the seed of the cocoa tree, it is one of the richest sources of anti-oxidants on the plant. A 100gram bar of dark chocolate with 70-85% cocoa contains 11 grams of fiber, 67% if the RDA for Iron, 58% of the RDA for Magnesium, 89% of the RDA for Copper, and 98% of the RDA for Manganese. It also has potassium, phosphorus, zinc, and selenium.

13. Eggs

Eggs are an excellent source of inexpensive, high quality protein. The egg whites contain over half of the protein, vitamin B2, B6, B12, vitamin D, as well as minerals such as zinc, iron and copper

14.Lean Beef

Meat has been getting a bad rep lately, but if prepared properly can yield an excellent return on nutrients. A three-ounce serving of lean beef contributes 50% if your daily value in protein. A high concentration of zinc, iron, and vitamin B-complex vitamins can also be found.

15.Cottage Cheese

Cottage cheese is a protein rich food that actually helps fight breast cancer. Another vitamin B-complex rich source, cottage cheese is heart-friendly and helps maintain blood sugar levels.

CARBOHYDRATES

Carbohydrates are among the main types of nutrients. They are the most vital source of energy

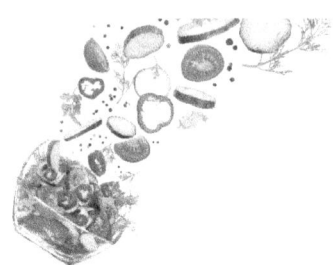

for the body. The digestive system alters carbohydrates into blood sugar (glucose). The body utilizes the sugar as the energy provider for the cells, organs as well as tissues. The body also stores any surplus sugar in muscles and in the liver for later use when it is required.

Dietary carbohydrates are split into 3 main categories:

Starches: They are long chains of the glucose molecules that ultimately break down into the glucose within the digestive system.

Sugars: They are sweet and short-chain carbohydrates which are found in various foods. Examples are fructose, glucose, sucrose and galactose.

Fiber: The human body lacks the ability to digest fiber. However, the bacteria found in the digestive system may use of some of consumed fiber.

GOOD VS BAD CARBOHYDRATES

The health benefits of good carbohydrates can be reaped by selecting the carbohydrates that contain lots of fiber. The latter carbs which get slowly absorbed into the body systems help to avoid spiking of the blood sugar levels. Few examples of good carbohydrates include; Vegetables, whole grains, beans and fruits.

The health risks of bad carbohydrates may be minimized by consuming fewer processed and refined carbohydrates which strip away the beneficial fiber. Few examples of bad carbohydrates include; white rice and white bread.

BENEFITS OF GOOD CARBOHYDRATES

The good carbohydrates play a major role in providing energy needed for the daily activities. The great benefits of good carbohydrates are;

1. Provide Energy

All activities require energy. Even simple activities such as walking and breathing need energy. The main energy source needed for the daily requirements is gotten from glucose. The source of this glucose is the sugars and starches that an individual eats. Sugars and starches break down into simpler sugar. This is facilitated by insulin during the digestion process. Glucose then enters into the cell wall. The surplus available sugar from food is stored in the liver, muscles, or other body parts. The stored carbohydrates are later converted into fat.

2. Filling Fiber

Fiber does not just regulate digestion; it also keeps one full for long time. The recommended amount for daily consumption of fiber is just 25-30, many meals that are plant-based offer much more and that means an individual will remain fuller for longer. For a meal that is super-filling, individuals should target 10-15 grams of the fiber from consumed foods and should try not to take meals which have less than 5 grams of fiber for optimum satisfaction. All the entire food sources of the carbohydrates are superb fiber sources as well. Fiber slows down the blood sugar so that one does not get hungry quickly. It also maintains the glycemic levels steady all day.

3. Nervous System Function

While the sugar makes an individual anxious and jittery, the complex carbohydrates help in providing the body a grounding effect and reduce nervousness and anxiety. It is the one of the main reasons why one may often get less stressed just after a having a bowl of oatmeal, a dish made of sweet potatoes or even a simple banana. Carbohydrates offer the body exactly what it needs all the through down to the body's nervous system. The carbs aid the body to produce a couple of enzymatic reactions as well as balance in every possible way.

4. Prevent Diseases

The fibrous food gives ammunition to the body for fighting given diseases such as obesity and type 2 diabetes. The fiber also helps in indigestion and keeps heart diseases and cholesterol under control. Fiber may be acquired from the whole grains and dietary fiber. Appropriate intake of calories and exercise control may also prevent numerous diseases such as the type 2 diabetes and other heart related issues. Low cholesterol carbohydrates may decrease or eliminate the heart related diseases.

5. Control Weight

The carbohydrates are often blamed for the gaining of weight. However, the fact is that they may help in controlling or decreasing weight if they are appropriately used. This entails proper choosing of carbohydrates which in fact helps an individual in early weight reduction. The appropriate diet of fruits, vegetables, and other fibrous foods help in weight loss. The diets which are rich in carbohydrates may be helpful in weight reduction as well as controlling of muscle.

Choosing Healthy Carbohydrates

Since the carbohydrates work in both ways by increasing and also reducing weights, there inclusion needs to be carefully done. This helps one in ensuring that carbohydrates are not responsible for their obesity. The following is a list of good carbohydrates that offer healthy contributions to the body.

· Fiber-Rich Fruits and Vegetables and Fruits

· Whole Grains

· Legumes

· Dairy Products that are low-fat

· Limit of the Added Sugar

· Beans

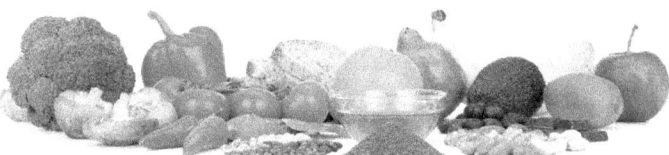

Carbohydr
ates make a vital part of an individual's diet, but it is recommended that their consumption should not be in large quantities. The carbohydrates are required for good health maintenance. Because energy is most readily available through carbohydrates, they should preferably make up around 40% of one's diet. Excesses are, however, always bad and the carbohydrates are not an exception. If the carbohydrates are excessively consumed, they may be harmful to health and may end up affecting the body in adversely. Some of the negative effects are;

1. Weight Gain

It is true that whole grains have more fiber and protein than the refined grains. The whole grains also have a slighter impact on the blood sugar levels and also promote control of appetite. Consuming the carbs that are primarily processed on the other hand has the opposite impact. The processed carbohydrates include; potato chips, soda crackers and cookies.

2. Insulin Resistance

Insulin is a hormone that the body releases to let the cells absorb blood sugar for energy storage. The carbohydrates that are more processed have greater impact on insulin and blood sugar levels according to research. As the level of insulin rises, the body becomes resistant to the hormone which results in high insulin and blood sugar levels that are long-lasting after eating. The Insulin resistance may cause type 2 diabetes and complications that are related to the type 1 diabetes. It may also contribute to a many serious health issues like heart disease, high blood pressure and even some types of cancer.

3. High Triglycerides

Triglycerides are a kind of fat found in the blood. If the levels become excessive, blood may be unable to freely travel through the arteries which may set-up heart attacks and other cardiac issues. A diet that is sugar-rich may raise the levels of triglyceride which risks for heart diseases.

4. Nutrient Deficiencies

Eating excessive processed carbohydrates leaves little room in one's diet for a nutritious fare, which increases the risk for mineral and vitamin deficiencies. The latter deficiencies may cause a wide range of symptoms which include poor hair, skin, nails and poor eye health, mood issues, headaches, concentrations difficulty and also fatigue.

BAD CARBOHYDRATES

- Soda

- Sugar

- White rice,

- White bread,

- White pasta

- Potatoes (which are typically complex carbs, but act like simple carbs)

- Pastries and desserts

- Artificial syrups

- Candy

It is indeed true that Carbohydrates have been flaunted as the feared food in trending diets. Also some of the Carbohydrates have been promoted as healthy nutrient sources that are associated with reducing the risks of chronic diseases. Thus, appropriate consumption is a very key aspect in benefiting optimally from Carbohydrates. Everyone can lead a healthy life if they consume the correct foods and the correct amount of food.

www.ingramcontent.com/pod-product-compliance
Lightning Source LLC
Chambersburg PA
CBHW072012280526
45788CB00005B/2019